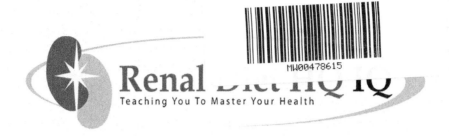

Renal Diet HQ IQ

Teaching You To Master Your Health

# Kidney Disease: Common Labs and Medical Terminology

## The Patient's Perspective

*By Mathea Ford, RD/LD*

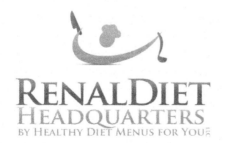

RENALDIET
HEADQUARTERS
BY HEALTHY DIET MENUS FOR YOU

# Purpose and Introduction

What I have found through the emails and requests of my readers is that it is difficult to find information about a pre-dialysis kidney diet that is actionable. I want you to know that is what I intend to provide in all my books. You can take this to fit a stage 2 – 5 kidney disease patient.

I wrote this book with you in mind: the person with kidney problems who does not know where to start or can't seem to get the answers that you need from other sources. This book will provide information that is applicable to predialysis kidney disease.

Who am I? I am a registered dietitian in the USA who has been working with kidney patients for my entire 15 + years of experience. Find all my books on Amazon on my author page: http://www.amazon.com/Mathea-Ford/e/B008E1E7IS/

<u>My goals are simple</u> – to give some answers and to create an understanding of what is typical. In this series of 12 books, I will take you through the different parts of being a person with pre-dialysis kidney disease. It will not necessarily be what happens in your case, as everyone is an individual. I may simplify things in an effort to write them so that I feel you can learn the most from the information. This may mean that I don't say the exact things that your doctor would say. If you don't understand, please ask your doctor.

I want you to know, I am not a medical doctor and I am not aware of your particular condition. Information in this book is current as of publication, but may or may not have changed. This book is not meant to substitute for medical treatment for you, your friends, your caregivers, or your family members.  You should not base treatment decisions solely on what is contained in this book.  Develop your treatment plan with your doctors, nurses and the other medical professionals on your team.  I recommend that you double-check any information with your medical team to verify if it applies to you.

In other words, I am not responsible for your medical care.  I am providing this book for information and entertainment purposes, not medical diagnoses.  Please consult with your doctor about any questions that you have about your particular case.

# TABLE OF CONTENTS

# YOUR KIDNEY TEST RESULTS – EXPLAINED

In this book, we will discuss the variety of medical and laboratory tests you may encounter as a person with kidney disease. It's very important to understand and know what your numbers are. You are the best advocate for your own health, and learning more about what you can do to keep your labs in the normal range is critical. Some labs tend to be low and some tend to be high when you have kidney disease. It can feel a bit like drinking from a fire hydrant – just too much information. However, you are going to learn and understand more and more when you know what you are looking at. Practice makes it easier to understand what you are doing to your kidneys one bite at a time.

Take this along with you to a medical appointment and write down your numbers. Or ask for a copy of your lab test results every time – your doctor shouldn't have a problem giving them to you. If they do, use a medical records request form to get a copy.

Remember that you are part of your kidney care team too! When you remove yourself from responsibility for your health, it only gets worse. Therefore, you need to be the one in charge. Take a notebook and write down the names of people who are involved in your care and you can call later with questions. Carry it with you. You are empowered to ask the questions that help you cope with your condition.

## TESTING YOUR DOCTOR DOES FOR CHRONIC KIDNEY DISEASE

Your nephrologist, or kidney specialist, checks urine and blood for chemicals that indicate how well your kidneys are working at that time. Your kidneys work 24 hours a day, 7 days a week, to keep your waste products from building up in your blood stream. Food and drink that you put into your body certainly affects the amount of waste in your body. This is why you have to eat a limited amount of protein and certain other types of foods.

When you watch what you eat, your labs will show it and you will feel much better and healthier. The chemicals that are measured in the blood and urine tests are parts of the foods you eat and the beverages you drink. Potassium, for example, is found in many fruits. So, when your body breaks it down the potassium is absorbed into your body and is part of your blood stream for your kidneys to remove.

In the next section, I am going to go over the most common lab tests and what they are used for, why they might be high or low – to help you understand what it might take to change the number in the right direction. Not to diagnose yourself, but to find questions to ask your health care provider.

You might wonder how you will know if your lab tests are normal. Each test has a normal range, usually printed on the results page and is based on that particular lab equipment. It will give a range that shows what is normal and if your number is outside that range it will indicate high or low. Each lab has it's own set of "normal" ranges because of the machines they use, so use the ranges given here as a guide, but ask your doctor about different ranges to make sure you understand where you are.

There are 3 types of blood cells.

1. Erythrocytes or red blood cells (RBC) - carry most of the oxygen and small amounts of carbon dioxide. Haemoglobin carries the oxygen molecule and gives blood its colour.
2. Leucocytes or white blood cells (WBC) - help fight infection as they can attack microorganisms.
3. Thrombocytes (platelets) - are parts of cells which plug small leaks in the walls of blood vessels and initiate blood clotting.

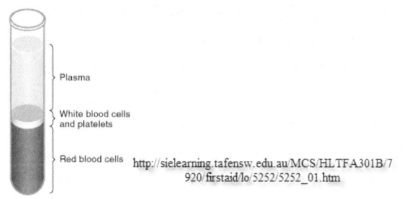

Plasma

White blood cells and platelets

Red blood cells http://sielearning.tafensw.edu.au/MCS/HLTFA301B/7 920/firstaid/lo/5252/5252_01.htm

Figure 1: Composition of blood

As you can see in the picture above, blood is made of several components. The red blood cells carry oxygen and are about 45% of the total volume of blood. White blood cells are a smaller amount of your blood, but do the very important job of fighting disease. They attack the foreign bodies in your blood and body to keep you healthy. Platelets are also a small part of your blood but they work to clot the blood when you get cut and stop your body from bleeding. Plasma is about 54% of the blood and helps the blood cells to float around in and make up the volume of blood. It carries many of the nutrients in the blood – your potassium, phosphorus, and creatinine for example.

Also, as it relates to terminology – some words that are used to describe levels of your lab results that you may have heard before. I want to remind you of what they mean.

**Hyper** means above or more than the normal amount. Hyperglycemia means high blood sugar. Hyperlipidemia means high blood cholesterol. If you see the word hyper added to another word, you can assume it means that it is higher than normal.

**Hypo** means the opposite – below or less than the normal amount. Hypoglycemia means low blood sugar. Remember these when your doctor is describing your lab result.

## Anemia

Anemia is a condition that causes tiredness and loss of energy, and is the result of a shortage of red blood cells to provide oxygen to the body's cells. People who are anemic typically feel cold and may be pale. It can cause headaches, dizziness, trouble concentrating and lightheadedness. You may experience other changes as well. When you are anemic, you may not heal as well and the lack of energy might keep you from doing your normal everyday activities.

Iron is a key factor in building your red blood cells. Hemoglobin has iron, and your body uses old, broken red blood cells to make new red blood cells in addition to the iron in the food you eat. If you don't have enough to start with, you will not have enough to make more red blood cells.

To test for anemia, your doctor looks at several lab results. Anemia can be very common for people with kidney disease, especially as it progresses toward dialysis. Once it is found, treatments can be started to get you back to a normal level of functioning again.

### Hemoglobin (Hgb) Levels
Hemoglobin is the oxygen carrying protein of your blood stream, and gives your blood its red color.

### Hematocrit (Hct)
Hematocrit is the percentage of your blood that is red blood cells. The more red blood cells you have, the more oxygen your blood can carry.

If either of these labs are high, you may be dehydrated. If they are low, it can indicate blood loss or anemia.

Both hemoglobin and hematocrit are important to let your doctor know if your red blood cells are functioning properly. But those are only part of the story. Your doctor may check another couple of labs if they suspect you have anemia.

FERRITIN

Ferritin is a lab that shows your doctor how much iron is stored in your body. While there are many types of anemia, iron deficiency is the most common. If your iron levels are low, you may be prescribed iron supplements to boost your body's stores and ability to make enough red blood cells.

TRANSFERRIN SATURATION (TSAT)

TSAT measures how much of your stored iron is available for your body to use to make new red blood cells. TSAT can be high with alcoholism or acute hepatitis, and can be low from chronic liver cirrhosis, malnutrition, iron deficiency, or chronic illness.

A drug that is sometimes used to increase the amount of red blood cells is based on a hormone that our bodies usually produce called erythropoietin (EPO). These drugs, called Procrit®, Epogen®, and Aranesp® provide the hormone (our kidneys normally make it but they find it difficult to do in kidney disease) that tells our bodies to make more red blood cells. So, if you have anemia, you need to increase the amount of iron available and then your body or a medication needs to tell it to make more red blood cells.

# Dyslipidemia

Dyslipidemia is an abnormal amount of lipids (fat) in the blood stream. The prefix dys means abnormal. Typically too much fat in the blood stream, but it can be too little as well. Because people can have heart problems as well as kidney disease, it is important to monitor those labs too! Your doctor is going to want to ensure you are getting the right kind of diet and keeping your cholesterol down.

Cholesterol is a soft, waxy fat in your blood that is used by your body to build cell membranes, insulate your nerve cells, and make hormones for your body. So your liver makes it because you need to have some. Another good thing to know is that your liver makes cholesterol – so any animal with a liver will make cholesterol. And plants will not have cholesterol. So, soybeans, wheat, and fruit do not have cholesterol.

Your cholesterol level has little to do with the amount of cholesterol that you eat and more to do with the amount of saturated and trans fat that you eat. These both turn into cholesterol in your body fairly quickly.

## Total Cholesterol

Goal for total cholesterol is less than 200 mg/dL for the general population. When testing cholesterol, you want to be fasting so that your doctor can get a good idea of the levels normally in your blood. Cholesterol goes up with eating because your body absorbs it from food and then processes it. Total cholesterol is a combination of the HDL, LDL, VLDL and triglycerides in your blood stream – although not a straight addition type of combination. The laboratory does a calculation to get to the total cholesterol number.

## HDL Cholesterol

HDL Cholesterol is the "good" cholesterol. It's the cholesterol that you want to have more of. I like to describe HDL cholesterol like garbage trucks, going around your body and picking up the extra LDL and triglycerides that are in your blood stream and returning them to your liver. So, you want more garbage trucks going around your body and picking up the bad "trash".

How do you get more HDL cholesterol? For the most part, it's exercise. Exercise will increase your HDL levels.

## LDL Cholesterol

Also known as the "bad" cholesterol, LDL is the cholesterol that is correlated with higher risk of heart attacks and stroke. It builds up in our blood vessels and leads to blockage. It can be decreased through the use of medication and dietary changes. Your physician will give you a target range, but with kidney disease you have a very high risk of heart attack so expect to need to keep it low.

VLDL means very low density lipoprotein, and is another type of the "bad cholesterol" that you want to decrease in your bloodstream. They are kind of an "in-between" form of cholesterol, and travel through the blood providing fat to your muscles, then once they are depleted of most of the fat, they are converted by your liver to LDL.

## Triglycerides

Triglycerides are the way that your body moves fat from being in your food to cholesterol in your body. Once you eat fat, it is encapsulated into a triglyceride and then your liver changes it into HDL, LDL, or VLDL. You know that your blood is mainly plasma (water), and you know that oil and water do not mix, so your body puts fat from your food into a form where it dissolves into the water until it can be processed.

Triglyceride levels are increased by higher levels of blood glucose and alcohol. If you are a diabetic and you have high blood sugar levels because of your body's inability to process sugar then your triglycerides are going to be high. This also increases your risk of heart attacks. So, decrease your triglycerides by decreasing the simple sugars in your diet and controlling your diabetes.

BLOOD PRESSURE
Ok, I will admit it – it's not a lab but it is related to your heart. And your doctor does check it. Keep it normal – less than 130/90 and you should be ok.

It can be measured at the drug store (most have the equipment where you can sit and put your arm in the cuff) or at home as well. You can purchase equipment for home use, and record your information to share with your doctor later. You can track it and see if certain days or activities raise your blood pressure so you can plan accordingly.

## ELECTROLYTE BALANCE

You may be wondering what an electrolyte is? Electro sounds like electricity – and that is what it is in many ways. The chemicals in your blood stream that carry the positive and negative "charges" around that your cells in your body needs are called electrolytes. Your body normally maintains electrolyte levels within a very specific range of numbers – and it does this for a good reason. Too much or too little of an electrolyte could cause a problem in your body. Healthy kidneys allow you to keep electrolytes in balance in your blood stream. As your kidneys become damaged, they are less capable of doing that.

### POTASSIUM

You may know a lot about potassium and your food. Now it's time to learn about potassium in your blood. Potassium allows your nerves and muscles to work – contracting and relaxing – including your heart. Having too little or too much can cause sudden problems and possibly death. Too much potassium in your blood (hyperkalemia) can make your muscles very weak and stop working. Too little potassium (hypokalemia) can cause tiredness, muscle weakness, paralysis and abnormal heart beating.

Kidneys manage potassium very well until they fail completely or are very close to failing. Making sure you are watching what you eat and asking about your potassium level keeps you in the know about any changes needed to your diet.

### CALCIUM

Calcium is a mineral you have heard about since you were young, I bet. Calcium is found in milk and many other things – we add it to a lot of foods like bread and orange juice. Calcium is important for your body to have healthy bones and muscle contraction. You might have taken a calcium supplement in the past to keep your bones healthy as well if you don't drink a lot of milk.

Your bones and teeth are where your body stores calcium it needs for your body functions. As your organs need calcium, your body removes small amounts from your bones.

Too much calcium in your blood is called hypercalcemia and can make you confused and irritable. Or put you into a coma. When you don't have enough calcium – hypocalcemia – you can have numbness, seizures, confusion or muscle spasms. You also could have long term problems with it damaging your bones related to hyperparathyroidism.

PHOSPHORUS

Phosphorus is plentiful in the world, and is contained in almost all foods that we eat. It's vital to your use of energy in your body. When labs measure the amount of phosphorus in your bloodstream, they refer to it as phosphate.

Phosphorus is stored in your bones just like calcium. Your body maintains a very strict level in your bloodstream and your healthy kidneys help to eliminate extra phosphorus from your body. Medications and a healthy diet can help keep down the amount of phosphorus in your diet.

When you have too much phosphate in your blood stream, you itch all over. Lots of people on dialysis complain about itching a lot and some of it is related to the phosphate levels in their blood. When you don't have enough phosphate in your blood, you can have muscle weakness and possibly a coma – but that is very rare.

One place many people get additional phosphorus in their daily meals is from food additives. Food manufacturers use phosphate additives to make their products creamier, juicier, and in general look good. Look for words that contain "phos" on the label for items to skip – remember the amount in the food items are listed in weight order – so the closer to the top the more the product contains.

The reason why phosphate binders work is the same reason your bones are strong. Calcium and phosphorus form a very strong bond in your bones and make the structure rigid. Phosphate binders are made from calcium and they draw in the phosphate in your food and bind with it in your digestive system – keeping you from absorbing the phosphorus. You eventually just pass it through as stool. Many people use antacids made with calcium like Tums®, but other drugs can also help that are prescribed by your physician. It's important to know your phosphate level and ask your doctor if you need to take any phosphate binders. Always take your phosphorus binders with meals.

SODIUM

Sodium is important for your body function as well. The balance of sodium keeps your blood from being too thick or too thin – because sodium attracts water and the right balance makes your blood just right in terms of thickness. It also helps your muscles to work properly. So you need sodium in your diet. But, if you don't have healthy kidneys your body has a hard time getting rid of the extra salt in your blood.

Salt can also raise your blood pressure and cause damage to the small blood vessels found in the kidneys over time. So it's important for you to limit your sodium intake.

Too much sodium in your blood results in hypernatremia, and makes you very thirsty, gives you headaches and raises your blood pressure. It can make your tissues swell with fluid and cause your body to hold water (known as edema). Not enough sodium, hyponatremia, can cause you to feel ill, nauseated, have muscle cramps and low blood pressure. If you have ever had water intoxication from drinking too much water and not eating enough when you are out in the hot sun, you might have felt this way.

## KIDNEY FUNCTION

Your doctor needs to know how well your kidneys are functioning. Your ability to remove the waste products from your intake and that your body makes tells your doctor what stage of kidney disease you are in. Your doctor may measure these tests yearly, quarterly, or monthly – depending on your condition. You should understand what they mean because it can be helpful to know what stage of kidney disease you are in.

### BLOOD UREA NITROGEN (BUN)

This sounds like a strange thing, and I will admit that at first, I was kind of surprised. But, it's truly the urea in your blood that makes the urine in your kidneys. What happens is this – when you eat protein, your body breaks it down and uses it for fuel. As your cells use it for fuel and building blocks to repair cells, the waste, called urea, is released into the blood stream for your kidneys to remove and form urine.

Your blood urea nitrogen level is then used as a gauge for how healthy your kidneys are and how good they are working to clean the waste from your blood stream. This is why we reduce the amount of protein that you eat as your kidneys become more damaged. So you reduce the amount of waste that is put into your blood stream for your kidneys to work with.

### CREATININE

Another waste product that your muscles produce is called creatinine. During the normal course of a day, your body uses energy and releases creatinine into your blood stream as waste. The more muscle you have, the more creatinine you make. It does not rely on the amount of anything that you eat, but the blood test does not account for differences in weight, race or gender.

### GLOMERULAR FILTRATION RATE (GFR OR EGFR)

GFR or eGFR (estimated glomerular filtration rate) is not an actual test that the lab does; it is a calculation of how well your kidneys are doing based on your creatinine level and your gender, race, and age. It is the standard by which your kidney disease stage is evaluated to determine how well your kidneys are functioning. Knowing your eGFR is critical to knowing what amount of restrictions you should have in your diet.

### STAGES OF KIDNEY FAILURE

Doctors use the eGFR number to determine which stage of kidney failure you are experiencing. As you progress in kidney failure, your diet changes. You should start to see a nephrologist about stage 3 to help control your related conditions and keep you from progressing to dialysis.

- **Stage 1** Normal (GFR > 90 ml/min)
- **Stage 2** Mild CKD (GFR = 60-89 ml/min)
- **Stage 3** Moderate CKD (GFR = 30-59 ml/min)
- **Stage 4** Severe CKD (GFR = 15-29 ml/min)
- **Stage 5** End Stage CKD (GFR <15 ml/min)

## Bone Conditions

You are at a higher risk of developing bone disease by having renal failure based on the levels of calcium, phosphorus and how your kidneys are working to remove the excess amounts of chemicals. These next few tests are to help you understand if you need to address the loss any further.

### Parathyroid Hormone (PTH)

You may know where you thyroid gland is – it's right in the middle of your neck covering your windpipe. On the back side of the thyroid gland are the parathyroid glands. These four glands control the amount of calcium in your blood. When your levels of calcium in your blood fall, they release parathyroid hormone which helps you increase the absorption of calcium from the food you eat and drink.

When you have high levels of phosphate in your blood, your PTH increases and pulls more calcium from your bones to counteract the increase in phosphate. This can, over time, cause damage to your bones and weaken them because you are not replenishing your bones with calcium.

## Blood Sugar Controls

If you have diabetes, you already know you need to test and track your blood sugar levels. It is very important to slowing the progression of kidney disease. When your blood sugar is high, it can affect the shape of red blood cells – and those misshapen blood cells can affect the very small blood vessels in the kidneys. The higher your blood sugar on a regular basis, the more problems you might have. Type 2 diabetes is the number one cause of kidney failure.

### Fasting Blood Glucose

Usually measured first thing in the morning after a 8-12 hour fast (not eating), the amount of sugar that remains in your blood stream is an indicator of your diabetes control. Most doctors recommend you keep your fasting number below 120 mg/dl. Discuss with your doctor if you have questions about your fasting numbers.

### HG A1C (FOR DIABETICS)

Now, if you have diabetes, you are already used to having your HbA1c checked. Called a hemogloblin A1c test, it is a measure of the average blood sugar over the past 2-3 months. What happens is that when your blood sugar is high, glucose (sugar) attaches to the red blood cells. Labs give this result as a percentage – so it should be below 7.5% for normal levels of blood sugar. If it is higher than that, it means that your blood sugar is normally running over 200 mg/dl, which can lead to long-term damage from diabetes to more than just your kidneys. Your doctor will check this every 3-6 months to make sure you are on track with your blood sugars over time. This is a report that tells your doctor how well you are "really" controlling your blood sugar levels.

## URINALYSIS TESTING

These tests are done on your urine instead of blood testing. They can show some things that your blood tests do not – like how much protein is getting out of your kidneys and into your urine.

### URINE ALBUMIN – TO – CREATININE RATIO (UACR)

This lab tests for kidney damage – a lower number is better. It is checking to see how much albumin and creatinine is in your urine. Instead of having to do a 24 hour urine collection, this test can be done with one sample and give a good indication of how much protein you are losing and your kidney disease status. And it's accurate even if you are a little bit dehydrated.

## MICROALBUMIN

When you have diabetes, you might recall having a microalbuminuria test done. This tests for very small amounts of protein in the urine, since damage happens over time and is important to catch early in the disease process to slow it down. Most of the time, when you have some amount of microalbuminuria, it can be treated with blood pressure lowering medications. If you have diabetes, your doctor should check for this one time a year at least.

## URINE ALBUMIN

Albumin is a protein that is in the blood stream, and can pass through your kidneys into your urine. Protein molecules are large, so if they are passing through the small blood vessels in your kidneys, then your kidneys are damaged – and the more that passes through the more damaged they are. Doctors sometimes refer to this as "leaky" kidneys. Doctors might use a dipstick to test for albumin.

## URINE HEMOGLOBIN

This test is done to see if red blood cells are passing through the kidney blood vessels and into the urine. This usually means damage to the kidneys or part of the urinary tract, so have it checked out right away.

## CREATININE CLEARANCE

Have you ever had to do a 24 hour urine collection – keeping the urine in the refrigerator is the grossest part to me! But anyway, when they do a 24 hour urine collection many times in addition to the amount of protein they test for, they will see how much creatinine (muscle wasting by product) is created.  Your blood sample tells the doctor how much creatinine you are making and the urine shows how much is being removed from the blood stream.  This is a very effective test to see how kidneys are doing overall.

## Protein – Energy Malnutrition

Checking for protein and energy malnutrition is an important part of keeping you in good health. Think about it – you might be tempted to eat very poorly and little amounts of protein to keep your kidneys in good health. But your body needs some protein, and it can't repair the day to day damage that is done when you don't eat enough. And not having enough calories and protein can lead to further problems and death. So, your doctor checks your level of a couple of nutrients to see that you are doing ok.

### Serum Albumin

Albumin in your urine is not a good thing, but that's because you need it in your bloodstream. The amount of albumin is very important and related to the amount of protein that is available in your body. It measures your overall nutrition for your doctor.

Malnutrition can lead to early death as you progress in kidney disease, so it's important to know how well nourished you are.

### Pre-Albumin

Pre-albumin is another measure of nutritional status. It's another blood protein that is good to know about but it can be affected by inflammation status. So, if you are sick or not doing well, and your levels are low, it might be because of the inflammation. Have it checked and track over time to know how well you are doing.

### C-Reactive Protein

C-reactive protein, also known as CRP, is a marker for your doctor to know your inflammatory process and status. If it's high, your labs are likely to be affected and he or she needs to help you manage your inflammation in your body to reduce your risk of other related events.

## OTHER LAB TESTING THAT YOUR DOCTOR DOES

### BICARBONATE
Bicarbonate measures the amount of acid in your blood, and can be affected by how quickly your body removes waste from the blood stream. This level can be corrected by medication that your doctor prescribes.

### VITAMIN D
Vitamin D is becoming a very important vitamin to patients. It can affect mood and depression, as well as other things. It is significantly involved in bone and heart health. Knowing your levels and if you have a need to supplement with an over the counter medication is valuable. Do not supplement unless your doctor instructs you to, as it can affect other medications and conditions. Many people are deficient just because they don't go out of the house enough or get enough direct sunlight. Have your levels checked out and see if you need additional amounts to improve your health.

# Helpful Hints For Dealing With Your Results

When you find out you have kidney disease, it is an overwhelming amount of information and may be a lot to cover. I hope that you have found this guide to be a good explanation of what labs to look at and how important all of them are.

## Start Tracking!

Now, you are tasked with knowing your labs and tracking them. You are following the proper diet, and when the changes happen in your labs, you want to be able to see where you were and where you are now. If your blood sugar begins to be in line and not high all the time, you will feel different. If you eat right (or just a lot better than before), you will see a change. And that should be something you are able to quantify. Mentally, you need that!

## Ask Questions When You Don't Understand

If one of your labs comes up different than you thought it should, ask your doctor or nephrologist. Even if you have come home and pulled out this guide, and thought that your labs should have changed but they did not or they went the wrong way – call your doctor and ask why. I know that seems strange, but it's invaluable to know what you need to do to change – and if it isn't producing the right results, you may want to do something different – or maybe it's just going to take a little longer.

## Know What You Have Changed

That said, track your changes. You should keep a small diary of the things that you have changed – on this day I ate out or no meat Mondays started, or something like that. It's very good to know when you made the change – trust me, you will forget and then you may wonder why it didn't improve when you have not been doing the change for long. (It always seems to take longer than it should!)

## Make Sure You Account For All Your Medications

Medications make a lot of difference in your kidneys. Medications are important for your health – but you might have a couple of options and one is bad for your kidneys. For example, ibuprofen and Tylenol are used for pain relief by many people. Ibuprofen and similar products are very bad for your kidneys, yet you might still be taking them without realizing they are damaging.

Take your meds to the doctor and have them look them over for any interactions or reactions with your conditions. Make sure your doctor knows all of the medications and over the counter pills that you take. The doctor can make changes or adjustments that will improve your kidney function without you having to do a darn thing sometimes. Awareness that you might be affecting your kidneys is the first step, then bring it to the attention of your doctors so they can make the changes you need.

GET YOUR PAST LABS AND COMPARE THEM
TO CURRENT LABS AND SEE HOW YOUR
CHANGES HAVE BEEN AFFECTING YOUR
HEALTH.